Letter to the Soviet Leaders

BY THE SAME AUTHOR

The Nobel Lecture on Literature
August 1914
A Lenten Letter to Pimen, Patriarch of All Russia
Stories and Prose Poems
The Love Girl and the Innocent
The Cancer Ward
The First Circle
For the Good of the Cause
We Never Make Mistakes
One Day in the Life of Ivan Denisovich

Aleksandr I. Solzhenitsyn

LETTER TO THE SOVIET LEADERS

New Preface by the Author

Translated from the Russian by Hilary Sternberg

PERENNIAL LIBRARY
HARPER & ROW, PUBLISHERS
New York, Evanston, San Francisco, London

A hardcover edition of this book is published by Harper & Row, Publishers, Inc.

LETTER TO THE SOVIET LEADERS. Copyright © 1974 by Aleksandr I. Solzhenitsyn. English translation copyright © 1974 by Writers and Scholars International Ltd. All rights reserved. Printed in the United States of America. No part of this book may be used or reproduced in any manner whatsoever without written permission except in the case of brief quotations embodied in critical articles and reviews. For information address Harper & Row, Publishers, Inc., 10 East 53rd Street, New York, N.Y. 10022. Published simultaneously in Canada by Fitzhenry & Whiteside, Limited, Toronto.

First PERENNIAL LIBRARY edition published 1975

STANDARD BOOK NUMBER: 06–080339–8

Author's Preface

This letter, with all the proposals it contains, was written before the KGB's confiscation of *The Gulag Archipelago* and was sent to the addressees six months ago. Since that time there has been no response or reply to it, nor any gesture toward one. Such is the secrecy in which our bureaucratic apparatus examines these matters that many ideas far less questionable than mine have vanished without trace. Nothing remains for me to do now but to make the letter public. The newspaper campaign against the *Archipelago* and the disinclination to acknowledge the irrefutable past might be considered as a conclusive refusal. But even now I cannot regard it as irrevocable. It is never too late for repentance; the way is open to all living creatures on this earth, to all capable of living.

This letter was born and grew out of a single thought: how to avoid the catastrophe with which we as a nation are threatened. Some of its practical proposals may cause surprise. I am prepared to withdraw them at once if someone offers not a witty critique but a constructive course of action, a better and, most important, fully realistic way out, with clear paths ahead. Our intelligentsia is at one in its concept of a desirable future for our country (the broadest possible freedoms), but it is equally at one in its total lack of action to realize that future. Everyone waits bewitched for something to happen *of its own accord*. But that something will not happen.

My proposals were offered, of course, with only the smallest grain of hope, but a grain nevertheless. A basis for hope does exist if only as a result of the "Khrushchev miracle" of

1955–6, that unpredicted, unbelievable miracle of the release of millions of innocent prisoners, combined with the threadbare rudiments of a humane legislation (although in other spheres other hands were simultaneously at work piling up the very opposite). This surge of activity of Khrushchev's went far beyond the bounds of political expediency; it was an unquestionably sincere impulse, essentially hostile to, and incompatible with, Communist ideology (which is why our leaders beat such a hasty retreat and moved methodically away from it). To deny the possibility that something of the sort may happen again means shutting out all hope for the peaceful evolution of our country.

March 1974

Letter to the Soviet Leaders

Introduction

I do not entertain much hope that you will deign to examine ideas not formally solicited by you, although they come from a fellow countryman of a rare kind—one who does not stand on a ladder subordinate to your command, who can be neither dismissed from his post, nor demoted, nor promoted, nor rewarded by you, and from whom therefore you are almost certain to hear an opinion sincerely voiced, without any careerist calculations, such as you are unlikely to hear from even the finest experts in your bureaucracy. I do not hold out much hope, but I shall try to say what is most important in a short space—namely, to set forth what I hold to be for the good and salvation of our people, to which all of you—and I myself—belong.

That was no slip of the tongue. I wish all people well, and the closer they are to us and the more dependent upon us, the more fervent is my wish. But it is the fate of the Russian and Ukrainian peoples that preoccupies me above all, for, as the proverb says: It's where you're born that you can be most useful. And there is a deeper reason too: the incomparable sufferings of our people.

I am writing this letter on the *supposition* that you, too, are swayed by this primary concern, that you are not alien to your origins, to your fathers, grandfathers and great-grandfathers, to the expanses of your homeland; and that you are conscious of your nationality. If I am mistaken, there is no point in your reading the rest of this letter.

I am not about to plunge into the harrowing details of the last sixty years. I try to explain the slow course of our history, and what sort of one it has been, in my books, which I doubt if you have read or will ever read. But it is to you in particular that I address this letter, in order to set forth my view of the future, which seems to me correct, and perhaps to convince you all the same. And to suggest to you, while there is still time, a possible way out of the chief dangers facing our country in the next ten to thirty years.

These dangers are: war with China, and our destruction, together with Western civilization, in the crush and stench of a befouled earth.

ONE

The West on Its Knees

Neither after the Crimean War, nor, more recently, after the war with Japan, nor in 1916, 1931, or 1941, would even the most unbridled patriotic soothsayer have dared to set forth so arrogant a prospect: that the time was approaching, indeed was close at hand, when all the great European powers taken together would cease to exist as a serious physical force; that their rulers would resort to all manner of concessions simply to win the favor of the rulers of a future Russia, would even vie with one another to gain that favor, just so long as the Russian press would stop abusing them; and that they would grow so weak, without losing a single war; that countries proclaiming themselves "neutral" would seek every opportunity to gratify us and pander to us; that our eternal dream of controlling *straits*, although never realized, would in the event be made irrelevant by the giant strides that Russia took into the Mediterranean and the oceans; that fear of economic losses and extra administrative chores would become the arguments against Russian expansion to the West; and that even the mightiest transatlantic power, having emerged all-victorious from two world wars as the leader and provider for all mankind, would suddenly lose to a tiny, distant Asiatic country, and show internal dissension and spiritual weakness.

Truly the foreign policy of Czarist Russia never had any successes to compare with these. Even after she had won the great European war against Napoleon, she did not extend her power over Eastern Europe in any way. She undertook to crush the Hungarian revolution—to help the

Hapsburgs. She covered the Prussian rear in 1866 and 1870 without gaining anything in exchange—that is, she disinterestedly advanced the power of the German states. They, on the other hand, entangled her in a series of Balkan and Turkish wars, where she lost repeatedly, and, despite her enormous resources and threatening gestures, she never did succeed in realizing the dreams of her leading circles to acquire the straits, although she entered her last (and for herself fatal) war with precisely this as her chief aim. Czarist Russia often found herself carrying out other people's missions quite unconnected with her own. Many of her foreign-policy blunders were the result of a lack of practical calculation at the top and a cumbersome, bureaucratic diplomatic service, but they also seem at times to have been connected with a certain streak of idealism in the thinking of her rulers, which hindered them from taking a consistent line in defense of the national self-interest.

Soviet diplomacy has rid itself of all these weaknesses, root and branch. It knows how to make demands, exact concessions, simply get things, in ways that Czarism never knew. In terms of its actual achievements it might even be regarded as brilliant; in fifty years, with only one large-scale war, which it won from a position no whit more advantageous than that of the other participants, it rose from a country riven by civil strife to a superpower before which the entire world trembles. There have been some particularly striking moments when success was piled on success. For instance, at the end of the Second World War, when Stalin, who had always easily outmaneuvered Roosevelt, outmaneuvered Churchill too and not only got all he wanted in Europe and Asia, but also got back (probably to his own surprise) the hundreds of thousands of Soviet citizens in Austria and Italy who were determined not to return home but who were betrayed by the Western Allies through a combination of deceit and force. No less an achievement than Stalin's have been the successes of Soviet diplomacy in recent years: for the Western world, as a single, clearly united force, no longer counterbalances the Soviet Union, indeed has almost ceased to exist. In finding the unity, steadfastness and courage to face the Second World War, and then the reserves of strength to pull itself out of postwar ruin, Europe appears to have exhausted itself for a long time to come. For no external reasons, the victorious powers have grown weak and effete.

At the peak of such staggering successes, the last thing a person wants to hear is other people's opinions and doubts. This, of course, is the worst possible time I could have chosen to approach you with advice or exhortations. For when outward successes come thick and fast, it is the hardest thing in the world to desist from piling up more, to place limitations on oneself and to change one's whole outlook.

But this is where the wise differ from the unwise: they heed advice and counsels of caution long before the need becomes overwhelming.

Furthermore, there is much about these successes that gives little cause for self-congratulation. The catastrophic weakening of the

Western world and the whole of Western civilization is by no means due solely to the success of an irresistible, persistent Soviet foreign policy. It is, rather, the result of a historical, psychological and moral crisis affecting the entire culture and world outlook which were conceived at the time of the Renaissance and attained the peak of their expression with the eighteenth-century Enlightenment. An analysis of that crisis is beyond the scope of this letter.

And something else one notices—and cannot fail to notice—about our successes is two astonishing failures: at the same time that we achieved all these successes we ourselves bred two ferocious enemies, one for the last war and the other for the next war—the German Wehrmacht and Mao Tse-tung's China. Circumventing the Treaty of Versailles, we helped the German Wehrmacht train their first officers on Soviet training grounds, where they received their first experience of the theory of modern warfare, tank thrusts and airborne landings, all of which later proved very useful to them when Hitler accelerated his military preparations.

And the story of how we bred Mao Tse-tung in place of a peaceable neighbor such as Chiang Kai-shek, and helped him in the atomic race, is recent history and very well known. (Are we not heading for a similar failure with the Arabs also?)

And here we come to the crux of the matter we are discussing: These failures stemmed not from mistakes committed by our diplomats, nor from the miscalculations of our generals, but from an *exact adherence to the precepts of Marxism-Leninism*—i.e., in the first instance, to harm the cause of world imperialism and, in the second, to support Communist movements abroad. In both cases *national* considerations were completely lacking.

I am well aware that I am talking to total realists and I shall not waste my breath on appeals such as: Oh, if only we could retrieve just a little of the bumbling idealism of the old Russian diplomacy! Or: Let's do the world a favor and keep our nose out of its business. Or: Let's take a closer look at the moral foundations of our victorious foreign policy—it brings the

Soviet Union power abroad, but does it bring any real benefit to her peoples?

I am talking to total realists, and the simplest thing is to name the danger of which you have a much more detailed knowledge than I, for you have already been looking uneasily in its direction (and rightly so) for a long time: *China*.

As our proverb has it: As the forest grew, so the ax handle grew with it.

In this case, nine hundred million ax handles.

TWO

War with China

I hope you will not repeat the mistakes made by many of the world's rulers before you: don't reckon on any triumphant blitzkrieg. You will have against you a country of almost a *thousand million* people, the like of which has never yet gone to war in the history of the world. The time since 1949 has evidently not been enough for the population to lose its high degree of fundamental industriousness (which is higher than ours is today), its tenacity and submissiveness; and it is firmly in the grip of a totalitarian system no whit less vigilant than ours. Its army and population will not surrender en masse with Western good sense, even when surrounded and beaten. Every soldier and every civilian will fight to the last bullet, the last breath. We shall have no ally in that war, none at least the size of, say, India. You will not, of course, be the first to use nuclear weapons; that would do irreparable damage to your reputation, which you cannot disregard, and anyway from a practical point of view still wouldn't bring you a quick victory. The opposing side, being more poorly equipped, is even less likely to use them. (And in general, fortunately, mankind is able to hold itself back from the ultimate brink of destruction by virtue of its simple instinct for self-preservation. Thus it was that after the First World War no one dared to use chemical warfare, and thus it is, I believe, that now after the Second no one will use nuclear weapons. So all the ruinously extravagant superstockpiling that is going on is senseless and gratifies only the scientists and the generals—this is the hard fate of those countries who have elected to be in the front ranks of the nuclear powers. The stockpiled weapons will never be of any use; and by the time the conflict erupts they will be obsolete.)

A *conventional* war, on the other hand, would be the longest and bloodiest of all the wars mankind has ever fought. Like the Vietnam War at the very least (to which it will be similar in many ways), it will certainly last a minimum of ten to fifteen years—and, incidentally, will run almost exactly along the lines forecast by Amalrik, who was sent to his destruction for what he wrote instead of being invited to join the inner circle of our advisers. If Russia lost up to one and a half million people in the First World War and (according to Khrushchev's figures) twenty million in the Second, then war with China is bound to cost us sixty million souls at the very least, and, as always in wars, they will be the best souls—all our finest and purest people are bound to perish. As for the Russian people, our very last root will be extirpated. And this will be the climax of a long line of extirpations, beginning in the seventeenth century with the extermination of the Old Believers, continuing with Peter the Great and a string of successors (which I will also leave to one side in this letter) and ending with this, the ultimate one. After *this* war the Russian people will virtually cease to exist on this planet. And that alone will mean the war has been lost *utterly*, irrespective of all its other consequences (for the most part dismal, including the consequences for your power, as you realize). One's heart bleeds at the thought of our young men and our entire middle generation, the finest generation, marching and riding off to die in a war. To die in an *ideological* war! And mainly for a dead ideology! I think *even you* are not able to take such an awesome responsibility upon yourselves!

One aches with sympathy for the ordinary Chinese too, because it is they who will be the most helpless victims of the war. They are held in such a strait jacket that not only can they not change their fate or discuss it in any way, they daren't even wiggle their ears!

This calamitous future, which is just around the corner at the current rate of development,

weighs heavily on us creatures of the present—
on those who wield power, on those who have
the power of influence and on those who have
only a voice to cry: There must never be such
a war. *This war must not happen, ever!* Our
task must be not to *win* the war, for no one can
possibly win it, but to *avoid it!*

I think I can see a way. And that is why I
have undertaken to write this letter today.

Why are we veering toward this war? For two
reasons. One is the dynamic pressure of a China
one thousand million strong on our as yet unexploited Siberian lands—not the strip that is now
being disputed on the basis of past treaties, but
the whole of Siberia—to which, in our scramble
for great social and even cosmic transformations, we haven't yet bent our energies. And
this pressure will increase as the earth becomes
increasingly overpopulated. But the main reason for this impending war, a reason that is far
more powerful and indeed is the chief and
insuperable one, is *ideological*. This should not
surprise us: throughout history there have been
no crueler wars and periods of civil strife than

those provoked by ideological (including, alas, religious) dissensions. For fifteen years now a dispute has been going on between yourselves and the Chinese leaders over which of you best understands, expounds and propagates the doctrines of the Fathers of the Progressive World View. And in addition to a fierce power struggle, there is this global rivalry developing between you, this claim to be the sole true exponent of Communist doctrine and this ambition to be the one to lead all the peoples of the world after you in carrying it out.

And what do you think will happen? That when war breaks out, both the belligerents will simply fly the purity of their ideology on their flags? And that sixty million of our fellow countrymen will allow themselves to be killed because the sacred truth is written on page 533 of Lenin and not on page 335 as our adversary claims? Surely only the very, very first of them will die for that....

When war with Hitler began, Stalin, who had omitted and bungled so much in the way of military preparation, did not neglect *that* side, the ideological side. And although the ideological grounds for that war seemed more indisputable than those that face you now (the war was waged against what appeared on the surface to be a diametrically opposed ideology), from the very first days of the war Stalin refused to rely on the putrid, decaying prop of ideology. He wisely discarded it, all but ceased to mention it and unfurled instead the old Russian banner—sometimes, indeed, the standard of Orthodoxy—and we conquered! (Only toward the end of the war and after the victory was the Progressive Doctrine taken out of its mothballs.)

So do you really think that in a conflict between similar, closely related ideologies, differing only in nuances, *you* will not have to make the same reorientation? But by then it will be too late—military tension alone will make it very difficult.

How much wiser it would be to make *this same* turnabout today as a preventive measure. If it has to be done anyway *for a war*, wouldn't it be more sensible to do it much earlier, *to avoid going to war at all?*

Give them their ideology! Let the Chinese leaders glory in it for a while. And for that matter, let them shoulder the whole sackful of unfulfillable international obligations, let them grunt and heave and instruct humanity, and foot all the bills for their absurd economics (a million a day just to Cuba), and let them support terrorists and guerrillas in the Southern Hemisphere too, if they like.

The main source of the savage feuding between us will then melt away, a great many points of today's contention and conflict all over the world will also melt away, and a military clash will become a much remoter possibility and perhaps *won't take place at all*.

Take an unbiased look: the murky whirlwind of *Progressive Ideology* swept in on us from the West at the end of the last century, and has tormented and ravaged our soul quite enough; and if it is now veering away farther east of its own accord, then let it veer away, don't try to stop it! (This doesn't mean I wish for the spiritual destruction of China. I believe that our people will soon be cured of this disease, and the Chinese too, given time; and it will not be too late, I hope, to save their country and protect humanity. But after all we have endured, it is enough for the time being for us to worry about how to save *our own* people.)

Ideological dissension will melt away—and there will probably never be a Sino-Soviet war. And if there should be, then it will be in the remote future and a truly defensive, truly patriotic one. At the end of the twentieth century we cannot give up Siberian territory, that's beyond all question. But to give up an ideology can only mean relief and recovery for us!

THREE

Civilization in an Impasse

A second danger is the multiple impasse in which Western civilization (which Russia long ago chose the honor of joining) finds itself, but it is not so imminent; there are still two or three decades in reserve. We share this impasse with all the advanced countries, which are in an even worse and more perilous predicament than we are, although people keep hoping for new scientific loopholes and inventions to stave off the day of retribution. I would not mention this danger in this letter if the solutions to both problems were not identical in many respects, if one and the same turnabout, a *single* decision, would not deliver us from *both* dangers. Such a happy coincidence is rare. Let us value history's gift and not miss these opportunities.

And all this has so "suddenly" come tumbling out at mankind's feet, and at Russia's! How fond our progressive publicists were, both before and after the Revolution, of ridiculing those *retrogrades* (there were always so many of them in Russia): people who called upon us to cherish and have pity on our past, even on the most Godforsaken hamlet with a couple of hovels, even on the paths that run alongside the railway track; who called upon us to keep horses even after the advent of the motorcar, not to abandon small factories for enormous plants and combines, not to discard organic manure in favor of chemical fertilizers, not to mass by the million in cities, not to clamber on top of one another in multistory apartment blocks. How they laughed, how they tormented those reactionary "Slavophiles" (the jibe became the accepted term, the simpletons never managed to think up another name for themselves). They hounded the men who said that it was perfectly feasible for a colossus like Russia, with all its spiritual peculiarities and folk traditions, to find its own particular path; and that it could not be that the whole of mankind should follow a single, absolutely identical pattern of development.

No, we had to be dragged along the whole of the Western bourgeois-industrial and Marxist path in order to discover, toward the close of the twentieth century, and again from progressive Western scholars, what any village graybeard in the Ukraine or Russia had understood from time immemorial and could have explained to the progressive commentators ages ago, had the commentators ever found the time in that dizzy fever of theirs to consult him: that a dozen worms can't go on and on gnawing the same apple *forever*; that if the earth is a *finite* object, then its expanses and resources are finite also, and the *endless, infinite* progress dinned into our heads by the dreamers of the Enlightenment cannot be accomplished on it. No, we had to shuffle on and on behind other people, without knowing what lay ahead of us, until suddenly we now hear the scouts calling to one another: We've blundered into a blind alley, we'll have to turn back. All that "endless progress" turned out to be an insane, ill-considered, furious dash into a blind alley. A civilization greedy for "perpetual progress" has now choked and is on its last legs.

And it is not "convergence" that faces us and the Western world now, but total renewal and reconstruction in both East and West, for both are in the same impasse. All this has been widely publicized and explained in the West thanks to the efforts of the Teilhard de Chardin Society and the Club of Rome. Here, in a very condensed form, are their conclusions.

Society must cease to look upon "progress" as something desirable. "Eternal progress" is a nonsensical myth. What must be implemented is not a "steadily expanding economy," but a *zero-growth economy*, a stable economy. *Economic growth is not only unnecessary but ruinous*. We must set ourselves the aim not of *increasing* national resources, but merely of *conserving* them. We must renounce, as a matter of urgency, the gigantic scale of modern technology in industry, agriculture and urban development (the cities of today are cancerous tumors). The chief aim of technology will now be to eradicate the lamentable results of previous technologies. The "Third World," which has not yet started on the fatal path of Western civilization, can only be saved by "small-scale technology," which requires an increase, not a reduction, in manual labor, uses the simplest of machinery and is based purely on local materials.

All the unrestrained industrial growth has taken place not over thousands or hundreds of years (from Adam to 1945) but only over the last twenty-eight years (from 1945 onward). It is this rapidity of growth in recent years that is most dangerous for mankind. The groups of scientists I mentioned have done computer calculations based on various possible courses of economic development, and *all* these courses turned out to be *hopeless* and pointed ominously to the catastrophic destruction of mankind sometime between the years 2020 and 2070 *if it did not relinquish economic progress.* These calculations took into consideration five main factors: population, natural resources, agricultural production, industry and environmental pollution. If the available information is to be believed, some of the earth's resources are rapidly running out: there will be no more oil in twenty years, no more copper in nineteen, no more mercury in twelve; many other resources are nearly exhausted; and energy and fresh water are very limited. But even if future prospecting uncovers reserves twice or even three times as big as those we now know about, and even if agricultural output *doubles* and man succeeds in harnessing unlimited nuclear energy, *in all cases the population will be overtaken by mass destruction in the first decades of the twenty-first century*—if not because of production grinding to a halt (end of resources), then because of a production surplus (destruction of the environment)—and this whatever course we take.

When everything is staked on "progress," as

it is now, it is *impossible* to find a *joint* optimum solution to *all five* of the problems referred to above. Unless mankind renounces the notion of economic progress, the biosphere will become unfit for life even *during our lifetime*. And if mankind is to be *saved*, technology has to be adapted to a stable economy in the next twenty to thirty years, and to do that, the process must be started *now, immediately*.

Actually, though, it is more than likely that Western civilization will not perish. It is so dynamic and so inventive that it will ride out even this impending crisis, will dismantle all its age-old misconceptions and in a few years set about the necessary reconstruction. And the "Third World" will heed the warnings in good time and *not take the Western path at all*. This is still perfectly feasible for most of the African and many of the Asian countries (and nobody will sneer at them and call them "Negrophiles").

But what about *us*? Us, with our unwieldiness and our inertia, with our flinching and inability to change even a single letter, a single syllable, of what Marx said in 1848 about industrial development? Economically and physically we are perfectly capable of saving ourselves. But there is a roadblock on the path to our salvation—the sole Progressive World View. If we renounce industrial development, what about the working class, socialism, Communism, unlimited increase in productivity and all the rest? Marx is not to be corrected, that's revisionism....

But you are already being called "revisionists" anyway, whatever you may do in the future. So wouldn't it be better to do your duty soberly, responsibly and firmly, and give up the dead letter for the sake of a living people who are utterly dependent on your power and your decisions? And you must do it without delay. Why dawdle if we shall have to snap out of it sometime anyway? Why repeat what others have done and loop the agonizing loop right to the end, when we are not too far into it to turn back? If the man at the head of the column cries, "I have lost my way," do we absolutely have to plow right on to the spot where he realized his mistake and only there turn back? Why not turn and start on the right course from wherever we happen to be?

As it is, we have followed Western technology too long and too faithfully. We are supposed to be the "first socialist country in the world," one which sets an example to other peoples, in both the East and the West, and we are supposed to have been so "original" in following various monstrous doctrines—on the peasantry, on small tradesmen—so why, then, have we been so dolefully unoriginal in technology, and why have we so unthinkingly, so blindly, copied Western civilization? (Why? From military haste, of course, and the haste stems from our immense "international responsibilities," and all this because of Marxism again.)

One might have thought that, with the central planning of which we are so proud, we of all people had the chance *not* to spoil Russia's natural beauty, *not* to create antihuman, multimillion concentrations of people. But we've done everything the other way round: we have dirtied and defiled the wide Russian spaces and disfigured the heart of Russia, our beloved Moscow. (What crazed, unfilial hand bulldozed the boulevards so that you can't go along them now without diving down into degrading tunnels of stone? What evil, alien ax broke up the tree-lined boulevards of the Sadovoye Koltso and replaced them with a poisoned zone of asphalt and gasoline?) The irreplaceable face of the city and all the ancient city plan have been obliterated, and imitations of the West are being flung up, like the New Arbat; the city has been so squeezed, stretched and pushed upward that life has become intolerable—so what do we do now? Reconstruct the former Moscow in a new place? That is probably impossible. Accept, then, that we have lost it completely?

We have squandered our resources foolishly without so much as a backward glance, sapped our soil, mutilated our vast expanses with idiotic "inland seas" and contaminated belts of wasteland around our industrial centers—but for the moment, at least, far more still remains untainted by us, which we haven't had time to touch. So let us come to our senses in time, let us change our course!

FOUR

The Russian Northeast

And here there is some extra hope for us, for there is one peculiarity, one reservation, in the arguments of the scientists I mentioned earlier. That reservation is: *The supreme asset* of all peoples is now *the earth*. The earth as open space for settling. The earth as the extent of the biosphere. The earth as a cloak over our deeply buried resources. The earth as fertile soil. Nevertheless, the prognoses for fertility are gloomy too: land resources averaged out over the planet as a whole, including any rise in fertility, will be exhausted by the year 2000, and if agricultural output can be *doubled* (not by the collective farms, of course, not by us), fertility, *on average for the planet as a whole*, will still be exhausted by 2030. But there are four fortunate countries still abundantly rich in untapped land even today. They are: Russia (that is not a slip of the tongue: it is precisely the R.S.F.S.R. that I mean), Australia, Canada and Brazil.

And herein lies Russia's hope for winning time and winning salvation: In our vast northeastern spaces, which over four centuries our sluggishness has prevented us from mutilating by our mistakes, we can build *anew*: not the senseless, voracious civilization of "progress"— no; we can set up a *stable* economy without pain or delay and settle people there for the first time according to the needs and principles of that economy. These spaces allow us to hope that we shall not destroy Russia in the general crisis of Western civilization. (And there are many lands nearer to us that have been lost through collective-farm neglect.)

Let us, without any dogmatic preconceptions,

recall Stolypin and give him his due. Speaking in the state Duma in 1908 he said prophetically: *"The land is a guarantee of our strength in the future, the land is Russia."* And on the subject of the Amur railroad: "If we remain plunged in our lethargic sleep, these lands will be running with foreign sap, and when we wake up they will perhaps be Russian in name only."

Today, because of the confrontation with China, this danger is spreading until it threatens virtually the whole of our Siberia. Two dangers merge, but, by a stroke of good fortune, a single way out of both of them presents itself: *throw away the dead ideology* that threatens to destroy us militarily and economically, throw away all its fantastic alien global missions and concentrate on opening up (on the principles of a stable, nonprogressive economy) the Russian Northeast—the Northeast of the European part and the North of the Asian part, and the main Siberian massif.

We shall not nurture hopes—we shall not hasten the cataclysm which is perhaps ripening, perhaps will even come to pass in the Western countries. These hopes may be deceived, just as the hopes for China were in the 1940's: if new social systems are created in the West, they may prove even harsher and more unfriendly to us than the present ones. And let's leave the Arabs to their fate, they have Islam, they'll sort themselves out. And let's leave South America to itself, nobody is threatening to take it over. And let's leave Africa to find out for itself how to start on an independent road to statehood and civilization, and simply wish it the good fortune not to repeat the mistakes of "uninterrupted progress." For half a century we have busied ourselves with world revolution, extending our influence over Eastern Europe and over other continents; with the reform of agriculture according to ideological principles; with the annihilation of the landowning classes; with the eradication of Christian religion and morality; with the useless show of the space race; with arming ourselves and others whenever they want it; with everything and anything, in fact, but developing and tending our country's chief asset, the Northeast. Our people are not going to live in space, or in Southeast Asia, or Latin America: it is Siberia and the North that are our hope and our reservoir.

It may be said that even there we have *done* a lot, built a lot, but we have done less of building than of destroying people, as it was with the "death road" from Salekhard to Igarka (but let's not go through all those prison camp stories again here). Building the railroad around Lake Baikal so that it became flooded, and sending the loop line senselessly through the mountains, so that the brakes burned, building things like the pulp mills on Lake Baikal and the Selenga River, the quicker to profit and poison—we would have done better to wait awhile. In terms of the speed of development in this century we have done very little in the Northeast. But today we can say: How fortunate that it *is* so little, for now we can do everything rationally, right from the start, according to the principles of a stable economy. Today that "little" is still fortunate; but in a very short time it will already be a disaster.

And what irony: for half a century, since

1920, we have proudly (and rightly) refused to entrust the exploitation of our natural resources to foreigners—this may have looked like budding national aspirations. But we went on and on dragging our feet and wasting more and more time. And suddenly now, when it has been revealed that the world's energy resources are drying up, we, a great industrial superpower, like the meanest of backward countries, invite foreigners to exploit our mineral wealth and, by way of payment, suggest that they carry off our priceless treasure, Siberian natural gas—for which our children will curse us in half a generation's time as irresponsible prodigals. (We would have had plenty of other fine goods to barter if our industry had not also been built chiefly on . . . *ideology*. Once again ideology stands in the way of our people!)

I would not consider it moral to recommend a policy of saving only ourselves, when the difficulties are universal, had our people not suffered more in the twentieth century, as I believe they have, than any other people in the world. *In addition to* the toll of two world wars, we have lost, as a result of civil strife and tumult alone—as a result of internal political and economic "class" extermination alone—66 (sixty-six) million people!!! That is the calculation of a former Leningrad professor of statistics, I. A. Kurganov, and you can have it brought to you whenever you wish. I am no trained statistician, I cannot undertake to verify it; and anyway all statistics are kept secret in our country, and this is an indirect calculation. But it's true: a hundred million *are no more* (exactly *a hundred*, just as Dostoyevsky prophesied!), and with and without wars we have lost *one-third* of the population we could now have had and almost *half* of the one we in fact have! What other people has had to pay such a price? After *such* losses, we may permit ourselves a little luxury, the way an invalid is given a rest after a serious illness. We need to heal our wounds, cure our national body and natural spirit. Let us find the strength, sense and courage to put our own house in order before we busy ourselves with the cares of the entire planet.

And once again, by a happy coincidence, the whole world can only gain by it.

Another moral objection may be raised: that our Northeast is not entirely Russia's, that a historical sin was committed in conquering it; large numbers of the local inhabitants were wiped out (but nothing to compare with our own recent self-extermination) and others were harried. Yes, it was so, it happened in the sixteenth century, but there is nothing whatsoever we can do now to rectify *that*. Since then, these spreading expanses have remained almost unpeopled, or even entirely so. According to the census, the people of the North number 128,000 in all, thinly scattered and strung out across vast distances. We would not be crowding them in the slightest by opening up the North. Quite the contrary, we are now sustaining their way of life and their existence as a matter of course; they seek no separate destiny for themselves and would be unable to find one. Of all the ethnic problems facing our country, this is the least, it hardly exists.

And so there is one way out for us (and the

sooner we take it, the more effective it will be), namely, for the state to switch its attention away from distant continents—and even away from Europe and the south of our country—and make the Northeast the center of national activity and settlement and a focus for the aspirations of young people.*

* Of course, a switch of this kind would oblige us sooner or later to withdraw our protective surveillance of Eastern Europe. Nor can there be any question of any peripheral nation being forcibly kept within the bounds of our country.

FIVE

Internal, Not External, Development

This switching of the focus of our attention and efforts will need to take place, of course, in more than just the geographical sense: not only from external to internal land masses, but also from external to internal problems—in all senses, from outer to inner. The actual—not the ostensible—condition of our people, our families, our schools, our nation, our spirit, our life style and our economy demands this of you.

Let us begin at the end, with agriculture. It is a paradox, impossible to believe: that such a great power, one of such military might and with such brilliant foreign-policy successes, should be in such an impasse, and in such desperate straits with its economy. Everything we have achieved here has been gained not by brains but by numbers, that is, through the extravagant expenditure of human energies and material. Everything we create costs us far more than it is worth, but the state allows itself to disregard the expense. Our "ideological agriculture" has already become the laughingstock of the entire world, and with the world-wide shortage of foodstuffs it will soon be a burden on it as well. Famine rages in many parts of the world, and will rage even more fiercely because of overpopulation, scarcity of land and the problems of emergence from colonialism. In other words, people cannot produce the *grain*. We, who should be able to, however, don't produce enough, or we shudder after one year of drought (and doesn't the history of farming tell us of cases of seven years in succession?). And all because we *won't* admit our blunder over the collective farms. For centuries Russia *exported* grain, ten to twelve million tons a year just before the First World War, and here we are after fifty-five years of the new order and forty years of the much-vaunted collective-farm system, forced to *import* twenty million tons per year! It's shameful—it really is time we came to our senses! The village, for centuries the mainstay of Russia, has become its chief weakness! For too many decades we have sapped the collectivized village of all its strength, driven it to utter despair, and now at last we have begun *giving back* its treasures and paying it fair prices—but *too late*. Its interest and faith in its work have been drained. As the old saying goes: Rebuff a man and riches won't buy him back. With the impending world-wide shortage of grain there is only one way for us to fill the people's bellies: give up the forced collective farms and leave just the voluntary ones. And set up in the wide-open spaces of our Northeast (at great expense, of course) the kind of agricultural system that will feed us at a natural economic tempo, and not flood us with Party agitators and mobilized labor from the towns.

I assume you know (it's obvious from your

decrees) about the state of affairs throughout our national economy and throughout our gargantuan civil service: people don't put any effort at all into their official duties and have no enthusiasm for them, but cheat (and sometimes steal) as much as they can and spend their office hours doing private jobs (they're forced to, with wages as low as they are today; for nobody is strong enough and no lifetime long enough to earn a living from wages alone). Everybody is trying to make more money for less work. If this is the mood of the nation, what sort of time-scale can we work to for saving the country?

But even more destructive is vodka. That's something else you know about, there was even that decree of yours—but did it change anything? So long as vodka is an important item of state revenue nothing will change, and we shall simply go on ravaging the people's vitals (when I was in exile, I worked in a consumers' cooperative and I distinctly remember that vodka amounted to 60 to 70 percent of our turnover).

Bearing in mind the state of people's morals,

their spiritual condition and their relations with one another and with society, all the *material* achievements we trumpet so proudly are petty and worthless.

When we set about what, in geographical terms, we shall call the opening up of the Northeast, and, in economic terms, the building of a stable economy, and when we tackle all the technical problems (construction, transportation and social organization), we must also recognize, inherent in all these aspects, the existence of a *moral* dimension. The physical and spiritual health of the people must be at the heart of the entire exercise, including every stage and part.

The construction of more than half our state in a fresh new place will enable us to avoid repeating the disastrous errors of the twentieth century—industry, roads and cities, for example. If we are to stop sweating over the short-term economic needs of today and create a land of clean air and clean water for our children, we must renounce many forms of industrial production which result in toxic waste. Military obligations dictate, you say? But in fact we have only *one-tenth* of the military obligations that we pretend to have, or rather that we intensively and assiduously create for ourselves by inventing interests in the Atlantic or Indian oceans. For the next half-century our only genuine military need will be to defend ourselves against China, and it would be better not to go to war with her at all. A well-established Northeast is also our best defense against China. *No one else on earth* threatens us, and no one is going to attack us. For peacetime we are armed to excess several times over; we manufacture vast quantities of arms that are constantly having to be exchanged for new ones; and we are training far more manpower than we require, who will anyway be past the service age by the time the military need arises.

From all sides except China we have ample guarantees of security for a long time to come, which means that we can make drastic cuts in our military investment for many years ahead and throw the released resources into the economy and the reorganization of our life. For technological extinction is no less a threat than war.

The time has also come to exempt the youth of Russia from universal, compulsory military service, which exists neither in China, nor in the United States, nor in any other large country in the world. We maintain this army solely out of military and diplomatic vanity—for reasons of prestige and conceit; also for expansion abroad, which we must give up if we are to achieve our own physical and spiritual salvation; and finally in the misguided notion that the only way to *educate* young men to be of use to the state is to have them spend years going through the mill of army training. Even if it is ever acknowledged that we cannot secure our defense otherwise than by putting *everybody* through the army, the period of service could nevertheless be greatly reduced and army "education" humanized. Under the present system we as people lose *inwardly* far more than what we gain from all these parades.

In reducing our military force we shall also deliver our skies from the sickening roar of aerial armadas—day and night, all the hours that God made, they perform their interminable flights and exercises over our broad lands, breaking the sound barrier, roaring and booming, shattering the daily life, rest, sleep and nerves of hundreds of thousands of people, effectively addling their brains by screeching overhead (all the big bosses ban flights over their country estates); and all this has been going on for decades and has nothing at all to do with saving the country—it is a futile waste of energy. Give the country back a healthy *silence*, without which you cannot begin to have a healthy people.

The urban life, which, by now, as much as half our population is doomed to live, is utterly unnatural—and you agree entirely, every one of you, for every evening with one accord you all escape from the city to your dachas in the country. And you are all old enough to remember our old towns—towns made for people, horses, dogs—and streetcars too; towns which were humane, friendly, cozy places, where the air was always clean, which were snow-clad in winter and in spring redolent with garden smells streaming through the fences into the streets. There was a garden to almost every house and hardly a house more than two stories high—the pleasantest height for human habitation. The inhabitants of those towns were not nomads, they didn't have to decamp twice a year to save their children from a blazing inferno. An economy of *non*gigantism with small-scale though highly developed technology will not only allow for but necessitate the building of *new* towns of the *old* type. And we can perfectly well set up road barriers at all the entrances and admit horses, and battery-powered electric motors, but not poisonous internal-combustion engines, and if anybody has to dive underground at crossroads, let it be the vehicles, and not the old, the young and the sick.

These are the sorts of towns that should adorn our frostbitten Northeast when it has been thawed out, and let that cosmic expenditure on space research be poured into the thawing-out process instead.

It's true that there was another special feature of the old Russian towns, a spiritual one which made life there enjoyable even for the most highly educated and which meant they didn't have to conglomerate in a single capital city of seven million: many provincial towns—not just Irkutsk, Tomsk, Saratov, Yaroslavl and Kazan, but many besides—were important cultural centers *in their own right*. But is it conceivable nowadays that we would allow any center of independent activity and thought to exist outside Moscow? Even Petersburg has quite lost its luster. There was a time when a unique and tremendously valuable book might be published in some little place like Vyshni Volochek— could our *ideology* conceivably allow that now? The present-day centralization of all forms of life of the mind is a monstrosity amounting to spiritual murder. Without these sixty or eighty towns Russia does not exist as a country, but is merely some sort of inarticulate rump. So here again, at every step and in every direction, it is *ideology* that prevents us from building a healthy Russia.

A man's mental and emotional condition is inextricably linked with every aspect of his daily life. People who are forced to drive caterpillar tractors or massive-wheeled trucks down grassy byways and country lanes ill-suited and unprepared for them, churning up everything in their path, or who, out of greed, jolt a whole village awake at first light with the frenzied revving of a chain saw, become brutal and cynical. It is no accident either that there are these innumerable drunks and hooligans who pester women in the evenings and when they are not at work; if no police force can handle them, still less are they going to be restrained by an *ideology* that claims to be a substitute for morality. Having spent a fair amount of time working in both village and town schools, I can confidently state that our educational system is a poor teacher and a bad educator, and merely cheapens and squanders the childhood and hearts of our young people. Everything is so organized that the pupils have no reason at all to respect their teachers. Schooling will be genuine only when people of the highest caliber and with a real vocation go into teaching. But to achieve this we will have to expend untold energy and resources—and pay our teachers much better and make their position less humiliating. At the moment the teacher-training institute has the least prestige of almost all the institutes and grown men are ashamed to be schoolteachers. School dropouts rush into military electronics like flies to a honey pot—is it really for such sterile pursuits that we have been developing these last eleven hundred years?

Apart from not getting what they need from the schools, our future citizens don't get much from the family either. We are always boasting about our equality for women and our kindergartens, but we hide the fact that all this is just a substitute for the family we have undermined. Equality for women doesn't mean that they have to occupy *the same number* of factory jobs and office positions as men, but just that all these posts should in principle be equally open to women. In practice, a man's wage level ought to be such that whether he has a family of two or even four children, the woman *does not need* to earn a separate paycheck and *does not need* to support her family financially on top of all her other toils and troubles. In pursuit of the Five-Year Plans and more manpower we have never given our men the right sort of wages, with the result that the undermining and destruction of the family is part of the terrible price we have paid for those Five-Year Plans. How can one fail to feel shame and compassion at the sight of our women carrying heavy barrows of stones for paving the streets or for spreading on the tracks of our railway lines? When we contemplate such scenes, what more is there to say, what doubt can there possibly be? Who would hesitate to abandon the financing of South American revolutionaries in order to free our women from this bondage? Almost every sphere of activity is neglected and in desperate need of funds, hard work and perseverance. Nor is *leisure* time an exception, reduced as it is to television, cards, dominoes and that same old vodka; and if anybody *reads*, it is either sport or spy stories, or else that same old idcology in newspaper form. Can this really be that seductive socialism-cum-Communism for which all those people laid down their lives, and for which sixty to ninety million perished?

The demands of *internal* growth are incomparably more important to us, as a people, than the need for any *external* expansion of our power. The whole of world history demonstrates that the peoples who created empires have always suffered spiritually as a result. The aims of a great empire and the moral health of the people are incompatible. We should not presume to invent international tasks and bear the cost of them so long as our people is in such moral disarray and we consider ourselves to be its sons.

And should we not also give up our Mediterranean aspirations while we are about it? But to do that, we must first of all give up our ideology.

SIX
Ideology

This Ideology that fell to us by inheritance is not only decrepit and hopelessly antiquated now; even during its best decades it was totally mistaken in its predictions and was never a science.

A primitive, superficial economic theory, it declared that only the worker creates value and failed to take into account the contribution of either organizers, engineers, transportation or marketing systems. It was mistaken when it forecast that the proletariat would be endlessly oppressed and would never achieve anything in a bourgeois democracy—if only we could shower people with as much food, clothing and leisure as they have gained under capitalism! It missed the point when it asserted that the prosperity of the European countries depended on their colonies—it was only after they had shaken the colonies off that they began to accomplish their "economic miracles." It was mistaken through and through in its prediction that socialists could never come to power except through an armed uprising. It miscalculated in thinking that the first uprisings would take place in the advanced industrial countries— quite the reverse. And the picture of how the whole world would rapidly be overtaken by revolutions and how states would soon wither away was sheer delusion, sheer ignorance of human nature. And as for wars being characteristic of capitalism alone and coming to an end when capitalism did—we have already witnessed the longest war of the twentieth century so far, and it was not capitalism that rejected negotiations and a truce for fifteen to twenty years; and God forbid that we should witness the bloodiest and most brutal of all mankind's wars—a war between two Communist superpowers. Then there was nationalism, which this theory also buried in 1848 as a "survival"—but find a stronger force in the world today! And it's the same with many other things too boring to list.

Marxism is not only not accurate, is not only not a science, has not only failed to predict a *single event* in terms of figures, quantities, time-scales or locations (something that electronic computers today do with laughable ease in the course of social forecasting, although never with the help of Marxism)—it absolutely astounds one by the economic and mechanistic crudity of its attempts to explain that most subtle of creatures, the human being, and that even more complex synthesis of millions of people, society. Only the cupidity of some, the blindness of others and a craving for *faith* on the part of still others can serve to explain this grim jest of the twentieth century: how can such a discredited and bankrupt doctrine still have so many followers in the West! In *our* country are left the fewest of all! *We* who have had a taste of it are only pretending willy-nilly....

We have seen above that it was not your common sense, but that same antiquated legacy of the Progressive Doctrine that endowed you with all the millstones that are dragging you down: first collectivization; then the nationalization of small trades and services (which has made the lives of ordinary citizens unbearable —but you don't feel that yourselves; which has caused thieving and lying to pile up and up even in the day-to-day running of the country—and you are powerless against it); then the need to inflate military development for the sake of making grand international gestures, so that the whole internal life of the country is going down the drain and in fifty-five years we haven't even found the time to open up Siberia; then the obstacles in the way of industrial development and technological reconstruction; then religious persecution, which is very important for

Marxism,* but senseless and self-defeating for pragmatic state leaders—to set useless good-for-nothings to hounding their most conscientious workers, innocent of all cheating and theft, and as a result making them suffer from universal cheating and theft. For the believer his faith is *supremely* precious, more precious than the food he puts in his stomach. Have you ever paused to reflect on why it is that you deprive these millions of your finest subjects of their homeland? All this can do you as the leaders of the state nothing but harm, but you do it mechanically, automatically, because Marxism insists that you do it. Just as it insists that you, the rulers of a superpower, deliver accounts of your activities to outlandish visitors from distant parts—leaders of uninfluential, insignificant Communist parties from the other end of the globe, preoccupied least of all with the fortunes of Russia.

* Sergei Bulgakov showed in *Karl Marx as a Religious Type* (1906) that atheism is the chief inspirational and emotional hub of Marxism and that all the rest of the doctrine has simply been tacked on. Ferocious hostility to religion is Marxism's most persistent feature.

To someone brought up on Marxism it seems a terrifying step—suddenly to start living without the familiar Ideology. But in point of fact you have no choice, circumstances themselves will force you to do it, and it may already be too late. In anticipation of an impending war with China, Russia's national leaders will in any case have to rely on patriotism, and on patriotism alone. When Stalin initiated such a shift during the war—remember!—nobody was in the least surprised and nobody shed a tear for Marxism; everyone took it as the most natural thing in the world, something they recognized as Russian. It is only prudent to redeploy one's forces when faced by a great danger—but sooner rather than later. In any event, this process of repudiation, though tentative, began long ago in our country, for what is the "combination" of Marxism and patriotism but a meaningless absurdity? These two points of view can be "merged" only in generalized incantations, for history has shown us that in practice they are always diametrically opposed. This is so obvious that Lenin in 1915 actually proclaimed:

"We are antipatriots." And that was the honest truth. And throughout the 1920's in our country the word "patriot" meant exactly the same as "White Guard." And the whole of this letter that I am now putting before you is patriotism, *which means* rejection of Marxism. For Marxism orders us to leave the Northeast unexploited and to leave our women with crowbars and shovels, and instead finance and expedite world revolution.

Beware when the first cannons fire on the Sino-Soviet border lest you find yourselves in a doubly precarious position because the national consciousness in our country has become stunted and blurred—witness how mighty America lost to tiny North Vietnam, how easily the nerves of American society and American youth gave way, precisely because the United States has a weak and undeveloped consciousness. Don't miss the chance while you've got it!

The step seems a hard one at first, but in fact, once you have thrown off this rubbishy Ideology of ours, you will quickly sense a huge relief and become aware of a relaxation in the entire structure of the state and in all the processes of government. After all, this Ideology, which is driving us into a situation of acute conflict abroad, has long ceased to be helpful to us here at home, as it was in the twenties and thirties. In our country today *nothing constructive rests upon it*; it is a sham, cardboard, theatrical prop—take it away and nothing will collapse, nothing will even wobble. For a long time now, everything has rested solely on material calculation and the subjection of the people, and not on any upsurge of ideological enthusiasm, as you perfectly well know. This Ideology does nothing now but sap our strength and bind us. It clogs up the whole life of society—minds, tongues, radio and press—with lies, lies, lies. For how else can something dead pretend that it is living except by erecting a scaffolding of lies? Everything is steeped in lies and *everybody knows it*—and says so openly in private conversation, and jokes and moans about it, but in their official speeches they go on hypocritically parroting what they are "supposed to say," and with equal hypocrisy and boredom read and listen to the speeches of others: how much of society's energy is squandered on this! And you, when you open your newspapers or switch on your television—do *you yourselves* really believe for one instant that these speeches are sincere? No, you stopped believing long ago, I am certain of it. And if you didn't, then you must have become totally insulated from the inner life of the country.

This universal, obligatory force-feeding with lies is now the most agonizing aspect of existence in our country—worse than all our material miseries, worse than any lack of civil liberties.

All these arsenals of lies, which are totally unnecessary for our stability *as a state*, are levied as a kind of tax for the benefit of Ideology—to nail down events as they happen and clamp them to a tenacious, sharp-clawed but dead Ideology: and it is precisely because our state, through sheer force of habit, tradition and inertia, continues to cling to this false doctrine with all its tortuous aberrations, that it needs to put the dissenter behind bars. For a false *ideology* can find no other answer to argument and protest than weapons and prison bars.

Cast off this cracked Ideology! Relinquish it to your rivals, let it go wherever it wants, let it pass from our country like a stormcloud, like an epidemic, let others concern themselves with it and study it, just as long as we don't! In ridding ourselves of it we shall also rid ourselves of the need to fill our lives with lies. Let us all pull off and shake off from all of us this filthy sweaty shirt of Ideology which is now so stained with the blood of those 66 million that it prevents the living body of the nation from breathing. This Ideology bears the entire responsibility for all the blood that has been shed. Do you need me to persuade you to throw it off without more ado? Whoever wants can pick it up in our place.

I am certainly not proposing that you go to the opposite extreme and persecute or ban Marxism, or even argue against it (nobody will argue against it for very long, if only out of sheer apathy). All I am suggesting is that you rescue yourselves from it, and rescue your state system and your people as well. *All you have to do* is to deprive Marxism of its powerful state support and let it exist of itself and stand on its own feet. And let all who wish to do so make propaganda for it, defend it and din it into others without let or hindrance—but outside working hours and *not on state salaries*. In other words, the whole *agitprop* system of agitation and propaganda must cease to be paid for out of the nation's pocket. This should not anger or antagonize the numerous people who work in *agitprop*: this new statute would free them from all possible insulting accusations of self-interest and give them for the first time the opportunity to prove the true strength of their ideological convictions and sincerity. And they could only be overjoyed with their new twofold commitment: to undertake productive labor for their country, to produce something of practical value on weekdays in the daytime (and whatever work they chose in place of their present occupation would be much more productive, for the work they do now is useless, if not positively detrimental), and in the evenings, on free days and during their holidays, to devote their leisure to propagating their beloved doctrine, reveling selflessly in the truth! After all, that is exactly what our believers do (while being persecuted for it too), and they consider it spiritually satisfying. What a marvelous opportunity, I will not say to test but to prove the sincerity of all those people who have been haranguing the rest of us for decades.

SEVEN

But How Can All This Be Managed?

Having said all that, I have not forgotten for a moment that you are total realists—that was the starting point of this discussion. You are realists par excellence, and you will not allow power to slip out of your hands. That is why you will not willingly tolerate a two-party or or multiparty parliamentary system in our country, you will not tolerate *real* elections, at which people might not vote you in. And on the basis of realism one must admit that this will be within your power for a long time to come.

A long time—but not forever.

Having proposed a dialogue on the basis of realism, I, too, must confess that from my experience of Russian history I have become an opponent of all revolutions and all armed convulsions, including future ones—both those you crave (*not* in our country) and those you fear (*in* our country). Intensive study has convinced me that bloody mass revolutions are always disastrous for the people in whose midst they occur. And in our present-day society I am by no means alone in that conviction. The sudden upheaval of any hastily carried-out change of the present leadership (the whole pyramid) might provoke only a new and destructive struggle and would certainly lead to only a very dubious gain in the quality of the leadership.

In such a situation what is there left for *us* to do? Console ourselves by saying "Sour grapes." Argue in all sincerity that we are not adherents of that turbulent "democracy run riot" in which once every four years the politicians, and indeed the entire country, nearly kill themselves over an electoral campaign, trying to gratify the masses (and this is something which not only internal groups but also foreign governments have repeatedly played on); in which a judge, flouting his obligatory independence in order to pander to the passions of society, acquits a man who, during an exhausting war, steals and publishes Defense Department documents. While even in an established democracy we can see many instances when a fatal course of action is chosen as a result of self-deception, or of a random majority caused by the swing of a small and unpopular party between two big ones—and it is this insignificant swing, which in no way expresses the will of the majority (and even the will of the majority is not immune to misdirection), which decides vitally important questions in national and sometimes even world politics. And there are very many instances today of groups of workers who have learned to grab as much as they can for themselves whenever their country is going through a crisis, even if they ruin the country in the process. And even the most respected democracies have turned out to be powerless against a handful of miserable terrorists.

Yes, of course: freedom is moral. But only if it keeps within certain bounds, beyond which it degenerates into complacency and licentiousness.

And *order* is not immoral if it means a calm and stable system. But order, too, has its limits, beyond which it degenerates into arbitrariness and tyranny.

Here in Russia, for sheer lack of practice, democracy survived for only eight months—from February to October, 1917. The émigré groups of Constitutional Democrats and Social Democrats still pride themselves on it to this very day and say that outside forces brought about its collapse. But in reality that democracy was *their* disgrace; they invoked it and promised it so arrogantly, and then created merely a chaotic caricature of democracy, because first of all they turned out to be ill-prepared for it themselves, and then Russia was worse prepared still. Over the last half-century Russia's preparedness for democracy, for a multiparty parliamentary system, could only have diminished. I am inclined to think that its sudden reintroduction now would merely be a melancholy repetition of 1917.

Should we record as our democratic tradition the Land Assemblies of Muscovite Russia, Novgorod, the early Cossacks, the village commune? Or should we console ourselves with the thought that for a thousand years Russia lived with an authoritarian order—and at the beginning of the twentieth century both the physical and spiritual health of her people were still intact?

However, in those days an important condition was fulfilled: that authoritarian order possessed a strong moral foundation, embryonic and rudimentary though it was—not the ideology of universal violence, but Christian Orthodoxy, the ancient, seven-centuries-old Orthodoxy of Sergei Radonezhsky and Nil Sorsky, before it was battered by Patriarch Nikon and bureaucratized by Peter the Great. From the end of the Moscow period and throughout the whole of the Petersburg period, once this moral principle was perverted and weakened, the authoritarian order, despite the apparent external successes of the state, gradually went into a decline and eventually perished.

But even the Russian intelligentsia, which for more than a century has invested all its strength in the struggle with an authoritarian regime—what has it achieved for itself or the common people by its enormous losses? The opposite of what it intended, of course. So should we not perhaps acknowledge that for Russia this path was either false or premature? That for the foreseeable future, perhaps, whether we like it or not, whether we intend it or not, Russia is nevertheless destined to have an authoritarian order? Perhaps this is all that she is ripe for today? . . . Everything depends upon *what sort* of authoritarian order lies in store for us in the future.

It is not authoritarianism itself that is intolerable, but the ideological lies that are daily foisted upon us. Not so much authoritarianism as arbitrariness and illegality, the sheer illegality of having a single overlord in each district, each province and each sphere, often ignorant and brutal, whose will alone decides all things.

An authoritarian order does not necessarily mean that laws are unnecessary or that they exist only on paper, or that they should not reflect the notions and will of the population. Nor does it mean that the legislative, executive and judicial authorities are not independent, any of them, that they are in fact not authorities at all but utterly at the mercy of a telephone call from the only true, self-appointed authority. May I remind you that the *soviets*, which gave their name to our system and existed until July 6, 1918, were in no way dependent upon Ideology: Ideology or no Ideology, they always envisaged the widest possible *consultation* with all working people.

Would it be still within the bounds of realism or a lapse into daydreams if we were to propose that at least some of the real power of the *soviets* be restored? I do not know what can be said on the subject of our Constitution: from 1936 it has not been observed for a single day, and for that reason does not appear to be viable. But perhaps even the Constitution is not beyond all hope?

Still keeping within the limits of strict realism, I do not suggest that you alter the disposition of the leadership which you find so convenient. But take all whom you regard as the active and desirable leadership and transform them *en bloc* into a *Soviet* system. And from then onward let posts in the state service no longer depend on Party membership as they do now. In doing so you can clear your Party of the accusation that people join it only to further their careers. Give some of your other hard-working fellow countrymen the chance to move up the rungs *without* having to have a Party card—you will get good workers, and only the disinterested will remain in the Party. You will, of course, want to keep your Party a strong organization of like-minded confederates and keep your special meetings conspiratorial and "closed" to the masses. But at least let your Party, once it has relinquished its Ideology, renounce its unattainable and irrelevant missions of world domination, and instead fulfill its national missions and save us from war with

China and from technological disaster. These goals are both noble and attainable.

We must not be governed by considerations of political gigantism, nor concern ourselves with the fortunes of other hemispheres: this we must renounce forever, for that bubble is bound to burst—the other hemispheres and the warm oceans will in any case develop without us in their own way, and no one can control this development from Moscow or predict it even in 1973, much less could Marx have done so back in 1848. The considerations which guide our country must be these: to encourage the *inner*, the moral, the healthy, development of the people; to liberate women from the forced labor of money-earning—especially from the crowbar and the shovel; to improve schooling and children's upbringing; to save the soil and the waters and all of Russian nature; to re-establish healthy cities and complete the conquest of the Northeast. Let us hear no more about outer space and the cosmos, no more historic victories of universal significance, and no more dreaming up of international missions: other nations are no whit more stupid than we are, and China has money and divisions to spare—let her have a try.

Stalin taught us—you and all of us—that *kindheartedness* was a "very dangerous thing," meaning that kindhearted rulers were a very dangerous thing! He had to say that because it fitted in with his scheme of exterminating millions of his subjects. But if you have no such aim, disavow his accursed teaching! Let it be an authoritarian order, but one founded not on an inexhaustible "class hatred" but on love of your fellow men—not of your immediate entourage but sincere love for your whole people. And the very first mark that distinguishes this path is magnanimity and mercy shown to captives. Look back and contemplate the horror: from 1918 to 1954 and from 1958 to the present day *not one person* in our country has been released from imprisonment as a result of a humane impulse! If the odd one has occasionally been let out, it has been out of barefaced political calculation: either the man's spirit was completely broken or else the pressure of world opinion had become intolerable. Of course, we shall have to renounce, once and for all, the psychiatric violence and secret trials, and that brutal, immoral bag of camps where those who have erred and fallen by the wayside are still further maimed and destroyed.

So that the country and people do not suffocate, and so that they all have the chance to develop and enrich us with ideas, allow competition on an equal and honorable basis—not for power, but for truth—between all ideological and moral currents, in particular between *all religions*: there will be nobody to persecute them if their tormentor, Marxism, is deprived of its state privileges. But allow competition honestly, not the way you do now, not by gagging people; allow it to religious youth organizations (which are totally nonpolitical; let the Komsomol be the only political one), grant them the right to instruct and educate children, and the right to free parish activity. (I myself see

Christianity today as the only living spiritual force capable of undertaking the spiritual healing of Russia. But I request and propose no special privileges for it, simply that it should be treated fairly and not suppressed.) Allow us a free art and literature, the free publication not just of political books—God preserve us!—and exhortations and election leaflets; allow us philosophical, ethical, economic and social studies, and you will see what a rich harvest it brings and how it bears fruit—for the good of Russia. Such an abundant and free flowering of inspiration will rapidly absolve us of the need to keep on belatedly translating new ideas from Western languages, as has been the case for the whole of the last fifty years—as you know.

What have you to fear? Is the idea really so terrible? Are you really so unsure of yourselves? You will still have absolute and impregnable power, a separate, strong and exclusive Party, the army, the police force, industry, transportation, communications, mineral wealth, a monopoly of foreign trade, an artificial rate of exchange for the ruble—but let the people breathe, let them think and develop! If you belong to the people heart and soul, there can be nothing to hold you back!

After all, does the human heart not still feel the need to atone for the past? ...

Perhaps it will seem to you that I have deviated from my initial platform of realism? But I shall remind you of my original assumption that you are not alien to your fathers, your grandfathers and the expanses of Russia. I repeat: the wise heed advice long before the need becomes overwhelming.

You may dismiss the counsels of some lone individual, some writer, with laughter or indignation. But with each passing year—for different reasons, at different times and in different guises—life itself will keep on thrusting exactly the same suggestion at you, exactly the same. Because this is the only feasible and *peaceful* way in which you can save our country and our people.

And yourselves into the bargain. For the hour of peril will come, and you will appeal to your people once more, not to world Communism. And even your own fate—yes, even *yours!*—will depend on you.

Of course, decisions like these are not made overnight. But now you still have the opportunity to make the transition calmly, over the next three years perhaps—or five, or even ten, allowing for the whole process. But that is only if you make a start now, only if you make up your minds this moment. For the demands life is going to make on you later will be even harsher and more pressing.

Your dearest wish is for our state structure and our ideological system never to change, to remain as they are for centuries. But history is not like that. Every system either finds a way to develop or else collapses.

It is impossible to run a country like Russia according to the passing needs of the day: in 1942 to condemn Nehru and his national liberation movement as a clique (for undermining the military efforts of our allies the English), and in 1956 to exchange kisses with him. And the same with Tito and with many, many others. To run a country like Russia you need to have a national policy and to feel constantly at your back all the eleven hundred years of its history, not just the last fifty-five—5 percent.

You will have noticed, of course, that this letter pursues no personal aims. I have long since outgrown your shell anyway and my writings will be published irrespective of any sanction or prohibition by you. All I had to say is now said. I, too, am fifty-five, and I think I have amply demonstrated that I set no store by material wealth and am prepared to sacrifice my life. To you such a vision of life is a rarity—but here it is for you to behold.

In writing this letter I, too, am taking upon myself a heavy responsibility to Russian history. But not to take upon oneself the task of seeking a way out, not to undertake anything at all, is an even greater responsibility.

A. SOLZHENITSYN